Herbal (Ayurved) Technique Weight Loss

(Eat Herbal Products and stay Fit.)

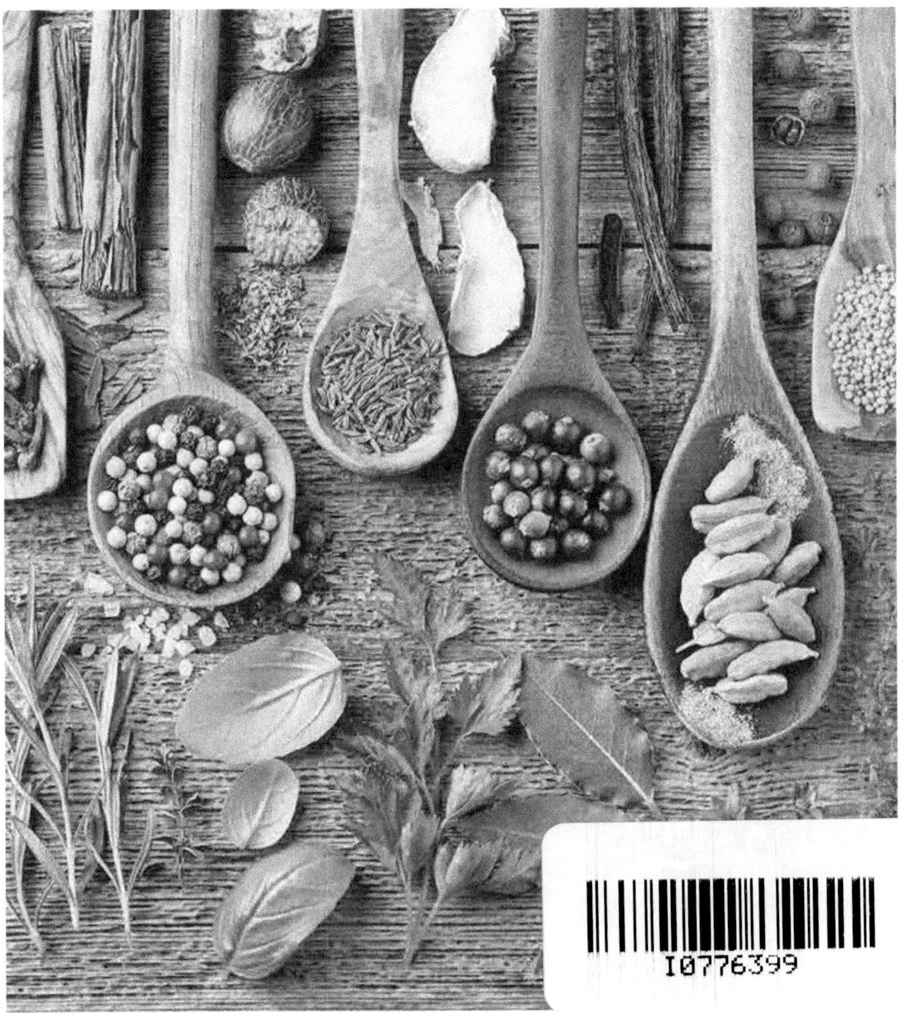

By; Shatrughan Ram

Herbal (Ayurved) Technique Weight Loss

Preface

2

You are on a diet yet your weighing scale is refusing to move? Does your diet stop at the sight of cupcakes, pizza, cheeseburgers, and potato crisps? To be honest, that's the case with most of us. I also cribbed about not losing weight even after being on a 'diet.' But then, I found out the real reason behind not losing weight. First, I was not following my diet correctly. Secondly, I needed to boost my metabolism and digestion to shed the fat. For this, a friend mine, who specializes in Ayurveda, recommended herbs and spices? So, I did my own research and gave it a try. And you won't believe, I lost three kgs in just one month! The best part, these herbs, and spices are easily available and cause no side effects. So ladies, if nothing is working out for you, try these 25 herbs and spices for weight loss and experience the change yourself! Let's begin.

Herbal (Ayurved) Technique Weight Loss

Index

1. Guggul Extract For Weight Loss

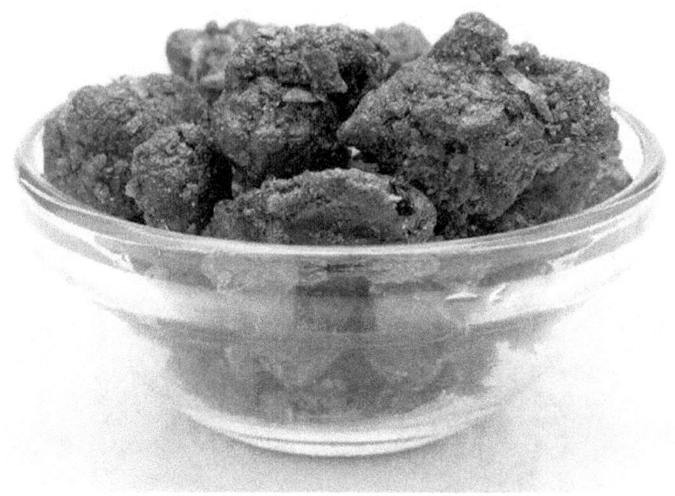

Guggul, also known as guggal, Devadhupa, Balsamodendrum Mukul, and guggulu sudha is the gum resin of Commiphora mukula, a native tree of India. It has been used in Ayurvedic medicine since ages. The guggul extract contains a phytosteroid called guggulsterone that has cholesterol lowering, anti-cancer, and anti-angiogenic properties. Guggul stimulates thyroid function, thereby boosting the metabolic rate and helping to burn the calories. Finally, guggul also contributes to lower levels of bad cholesterol (LDL cholesterol) and therefore is used for treating atherosclerosis.

Where To Buy Guggul?

You can buy guggul from any pharmacy or Ayurveda store.

How To Take Guggul For Weight Loss?

Consult your doctor before taking this Ayurvedic medicine.

- Typically, 25 mg guggul thrice a day is recommended.
- Keep 1 gm or ¼ teaspoon of guggul under your tongue and let it dissolve slowly. You can do this 3-4 times a day.

Guggul Weight Loss Recipe

- ¼ teaspoon guggul extract
- ½ cup water
- ½ teaspoon triphala powder
- Dissolve guggul and triphala in ½ cup of water.
- Let is soak overnight.
- Strain and drink the water in the morning.

Benefits

A combination of guggul and triphala is ideal if you are trying to lose weight. Guggul helps to regulate the thyroid hormone, boosts metabolism, and lowers bad cholesterol. Triphala improves digestion, cleanses the colon, and has antioxidant properties.

<u>**Precautions**</u>

Do not consume if your doctor doesn't recommend it. Avoid an overdose as it is likely to cause nausea, vomiting, and diarrhea.

2. Ginseng For Weight Loss

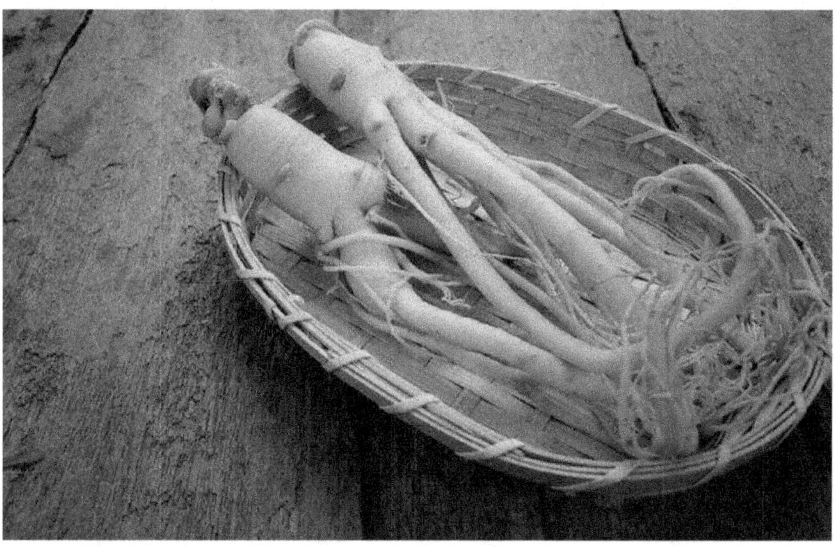

Ginseng is a slow-growing perennial plant that has fleshy roots. This plant mostly grows in cooler regions such as China, Bhutan, North America, Korea, and eastern Siberia. It has been used as a medicine by the Chinese for centuries. Research shows that ginseng can be used to treat stress, diabetes, lower cholesterol, and regulate blood sugar levels. Stress, unregulated blood sugar, and high cholesterol are all contributors to bad health and weight gain. Ginseng also helps to boost your metabolism and keeps your energy levels high throughout the day. Therefore, drinking ginseng tea will take care of the leading causes of weight gain.

Where To Buy Ginseng?

You can buy ginseng online or in any pharmacy and Ayurveda stores.

How To Take Ginseng For Weight Loss?

- 5 gm ginseng extract twice a day. You can reduce the amount to 2 gm after 2 weeks.
- 15-25 drops of ginseng extract in your tea or water twice a day.

Ginseng Tea Weight Loss Recipe

Ingredients

- 3 tablespoon ginseng extract
- 500 ml water
- 1 tablespoon lime juice
- ½ teaspoon cinnamon powder

How To Prepare

1. Boil water in a pan and let it cool for 5 minutes.
2. Add the ginseng extract and let it steep for 5 minutes.
3. Strain the water and add lime juice and cinnamon powder.
4. Stir well before drinking.

<u>Benefits</u>

Ginseng extract will help you relax, boost your energy levels and metabolic rate, lower cholesterol and regulate blood sugar levels. Cinnamon also aids weight loss by lowering bad cholesterol levels and lowering blood pressure. Lime is a storehouse of vitamin C that helps boost the immunity, and it is also rich in fiber that helps to reduce appetite.

<u>Precautions</u>

Do not overdose and immediately seek medical attention if you develop an allergy after consuming ginseng.

3. Hibiscus Tea For Weight Loss

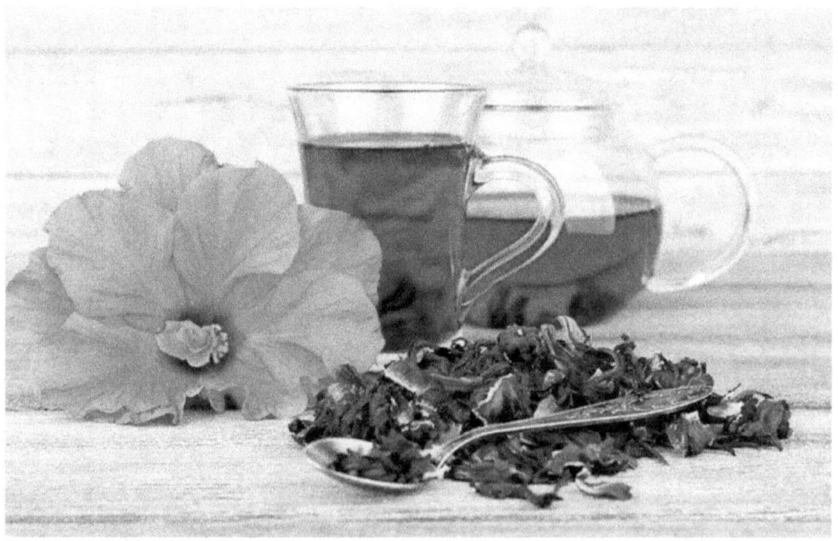

Hibiscus tea, the vermillion colored hibiscus flower extract, helps in weight loss by getting rid of excess water in the body. Hibiscus has diuretic properties and helps to prevent bloating. It contains an enzyme called, phaseolamin that inhibits the production of another enzyme, amylase. Amylase helps to break down carbs into sugar molecules. And therefore by limiting the production of amylase, phaseolamin reduces carb absorption by the body. Moreover, hibiscus tea is low in calories and increases satiety.

Where To Buy Hibiscus Tea?

You can buy hibiscus tea in supermarkets, online stores, and pharmacies.

How To Take Hibiscus Tea For Weight Loss?

1 cup hibiscus tea contains approximately 1.5 g hibiscus calyx. You can have 2 cups of hibiscus tea per day.

Hibiscus Tea Weight Loss Recipe

Ingredients

- 2 teaspoons of dried hibiscus flowers
- 2 cups water
- 1 teaspoon honey

How To Prepare

1. Put the dried hibiscus flowers into a teapot.
2. Boil 2 cups of water and pour it into the teapot.

3. Let it steep for 5-6 minutes.

4. Strain a cup of hibiscus tea.

5. Add honey and stir well.

Benefits

Hibiscus tea helps prevent irritation in the stomach, has diuretic properties, lowers cholesterol, and improves bowel movement. Honey is useful against throat infections, gastrointestinal disorders, and regulates blood sugar levels. Good gut health, low cholesterol, and an improved immune system aid weight loss.

4. Yerba Mate for Weight Loss

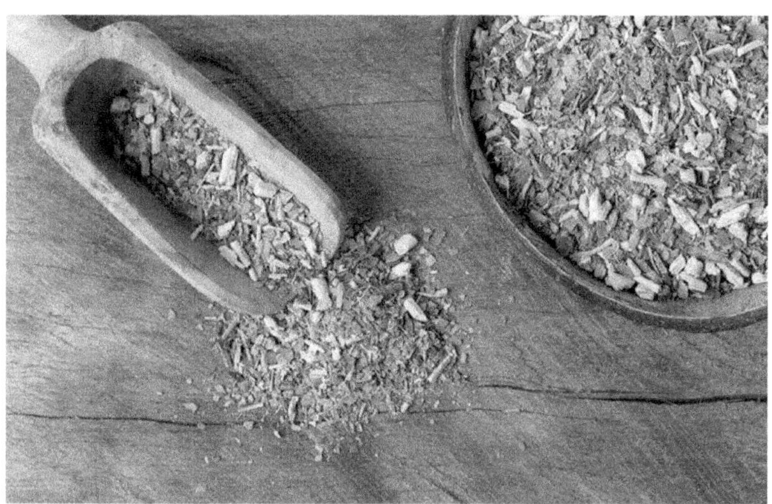

Yerba mate, a traditional South American drink, is made of aged and dried yerba mate plant. It is one of the ingredients of energy drinks in the market. Yerba mate contains polyphenols and three xanthines, caffeine being one of the xanthines. Yerba mate has been found to possess blood sugar lowering properties

Herbal (Ayurved) Technique Weight Loss

and also helps reduce the risk of diabetes mellitus. It also contains phytonutrients that help boost mood, keeps the energy levels high, suppresses appetite and aids weight loss.

Where To Buy Yerba Mate?

You can buy yerba mate in online stores.

How To Take Yerba Mate For Weight Loss?

You can take 10 g yerba mate and consume it as tea. Take hibiscus tea twice daily for effective results.

Yerba Mate Weight Loss Recipe

Ingredients

- 1 tablespoon aged and dried yerba mate
- 2 cups water

How To Prepare

1. Put 1 tablespoon yerba mate into a teapot.
2. Bring 2 cups of water to a boil.
3. Add the boiling water into the teapot.
4. Let it steep for 5 minutes.
5. Strain the yerba mate tea into a cup.

One of the best ways to lose weight effectively is to drink yerba mate tea. It keeps your energy levels high, and therefore you have the energy to workout or go for a walk to expend the energy. It suppresses appetite and keeps the stress away, which directly promotes weight loss.

5. Green Tea For Weight Loss

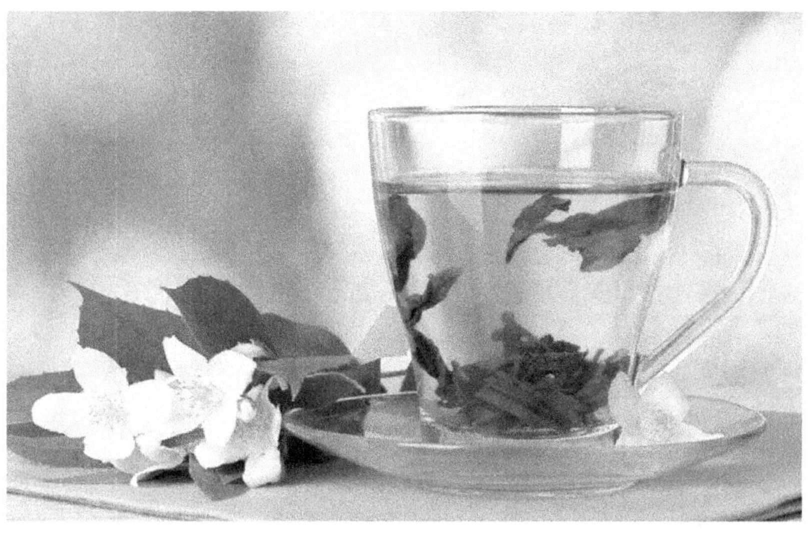

Undoubtedly green tea is always the best herbal tea for weight loss. It is rich in antioxidants called catechins. One of the catechins known as the Epigallocatechin gallate is a metabolism booster. Also, though green tea contains caffeine in lesser amounts when compared to coffee, caffeine helps to stimulate fat burning and better muscle performance. Green tea is also an excellent appetite suppressor which will curb cravings and make you eat less if you consume it 30 minutes before a meal.

Where To Buy Green Tea?

You can buy green tea from a local supermarket or online.

How To Take Green Tea For Weight Loss?

It is best that you use the green tea leaves to prepare a cup of tea. You can have as many as 4 cups of green tea per day. The best way is to drink a cup of green tea 20-30 minutes before a meal.

Green Tea Weight Loss Recipe

Ingredients

- 2 teaspoons green tea leaves
- 1 cup water
- ¼ teaspoon cinnamon

How To Prepare

1. Bring a cup of water to a boil.
2. Add the cinnamon powder and simmer for 2 minutes.
3. Turn the flame off and add the green tea leaves.
4. Let it steep for 5-7 minutes.
5. Strain and stir well before drinking.

Benefits

Green tea and cinnamon are powerful weight loss agents. Green tea boosts metabolism and melts fat. Cinnamon aids weight loss by regulating the blood sugar levels, insulin levels, lowering cholesterol, and suppressing appetite.

Precautions

Do not drink too much green tea as it may lead to insomnia, diarrhea, vomiting, heartburn, and dizziness.

6. Pu-erh Tea For Weight Loss

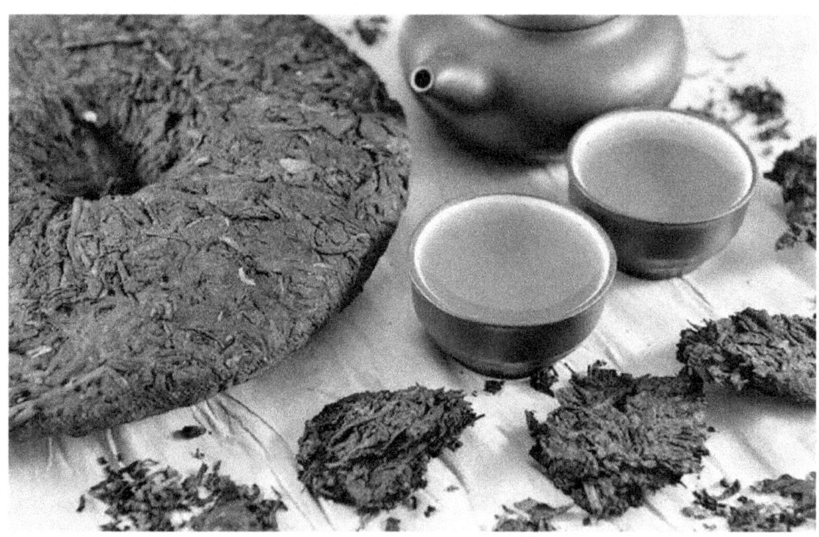

Pu-erh Tea, named after the city Pu-erh in China is a fermented tea. The tea leaves are first dried and rolled before being fermented and oxidized by microbes. Like wine, these tea leaves are left to age to add flavor and taste to the tea. The Pu-erh tea acts by keeping the spleen healthy and thereby helping proper digestion and absorption. This, in turn, accelerates the metabolic rate that leads to weight loss.

Where To Buy Pu-erh Tea?

You can buy Pu-erh Tea online.

How To Take Pu-erh Tea?

Take 1 cup of Pu-erh Tea after breakfast, lunch, and dinner.

Pu-erh Tea Weight Loss Recipe

Ingredients

- 1 teaspoon Pu-erh tea leaves
- 1 cup water

How To Prepare

1. Put Pu-erh tea leaves in a teapot.
2. Use a few drops of hot water to rinse the Pu-erh tea leaves.
3. Now, bring the cup of water to a boil.
4. Pour the boiled water into the teapot containing Pu-erh tea leaves.
5. Let it steep for 5 minutes.
6. Strain before drinking.

<u>**Benefits**</u>

Drinking Pu-erh tea will help boost your metabolism. It will also help keep your gut healthy and support better bowel movement. You will be able to burn and mobilize fat, which is essential if you want to lose weight.

<u>**Precautions**</u>

Do not drink Pu-erh tea before meals, as you will gain weight instead of losing. An overdose of this can lead to irregular heartbeats, irritability, ringing ears, and confusion.

7. Coleus Forskohlii For Weight Loss

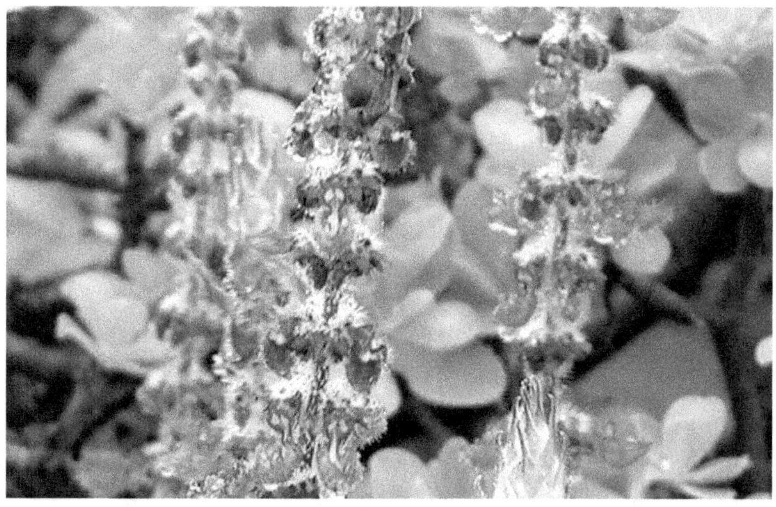

Coleus forskohlii, also known as Indian coleus is native to Southern Asia. Its roots are used in pickles and help to strengthen heart muscles. The roots have been used since ages as an Ayurvedic medicine. Coleus' roots contain forskohlin that stimulates the thyroid. It also helps to generate ATP which is why you will feel more energetic after consuming the root. Also, in males, it stimulates testosterone production, which helps to build lean muscle mass.

Where To Buy Coleus Forskohlii?

You can buy Coleus Forskohlii from Ayurveda stores or online.

How To Take Coleus Forskohlii?

You can have Coleus' root pickle or the extract that contains 18% forskohlin. You can have 50 mg of Coleus twice a day.

Coleus Forskohlii Weight Loss Recipe

Ingredients

- 1 Coleus soft gel
- 1 cup water
- 1 teaspoon lime juice

How To Prepare

1. Puncture the soft gel and take out the coleus extract.
2. Add it to a cup of cold water.
3. Add lime and stir well.

Benefits

Lime and coleus forskohlii is a unique combination but both works to help reduce weight. This drink will keep you active and energetic all day long. This will also improve your muscle and brain function. Your metabolism and immunity will also be boosted.

Precautions

Avoid taking this supplement if you are pregnant or are a breastfeeding mother. Overdose can also cause bleeding problems and low blood pressure.

8. Gurmar Leaves For Weight Loss

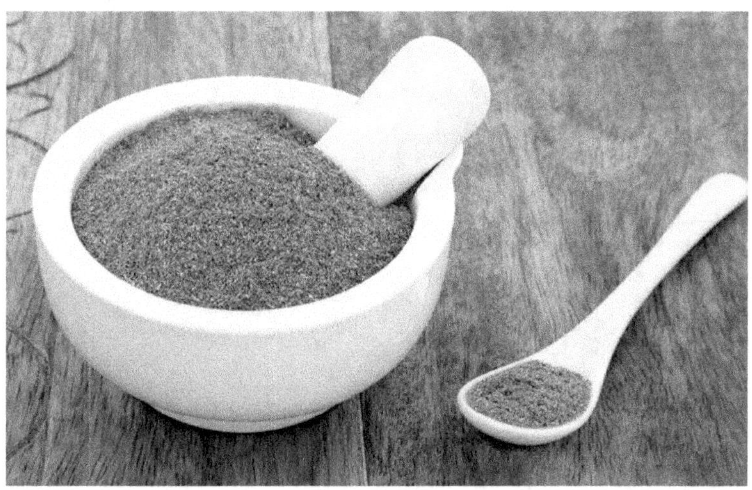

Gurmar is a perennial climber, mostly found in India and Sri Lanka, has oval leaves and bears yellow flowers. This herb is well known in Ayurveda as it has been used for centuries to treat kidney stones, obesity, diabetes, and constipation. This herb contains a compound called the gymnemic acid that prevents sugar absorption in the intestine and increases insulin sensitivity.

Where To Buy Gurmar Leaves?

You can buy it online or in Ayurveda stores.

How To Take Gurmar Leaves?

Gurmar leaves are available in powdered form, which you can take 400 mg per day. If you opt for dry leaf, you can take 1-2 gms per day.

Gurmar Weight Loss Recipe

Ingredients

- 1 teaspoon gurmar powder
- 1 cup warm water
- 1 teaspoon honey

How To Prepare

1. Add the gurmar powder to a cup of warm water.
2. Let it steep for 5-7 minutes.
3. Strain and add honey.
4. Stir well before drinking.

Benefits

The combination of Gurmar honey works wonders for weight loss. Since gurmar is a little bitter in taste, honey helps to sweeten it. Also, honey is loaded with antibacterial, antioxidant, and wound healing properties. It helps to regulate the blood sugar levels.

Precautions

Should not be taken during pregnancy and breastfeeding period. Stop using gurmar two weeks before a surgery.

9. Aloe Vera For Weight Loss

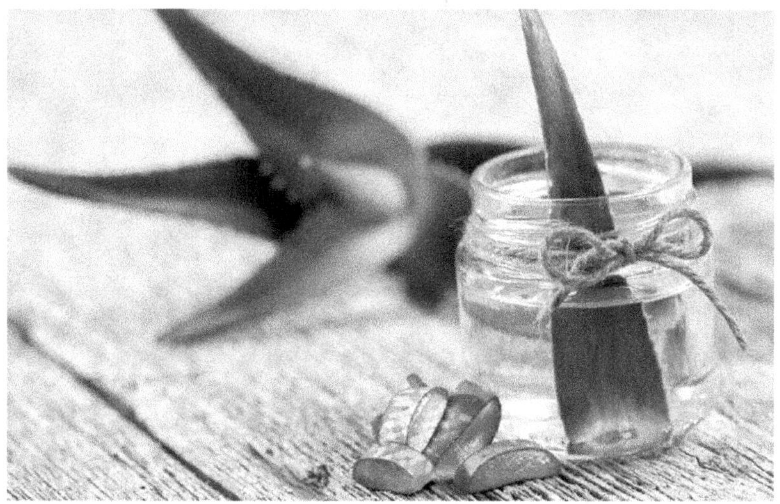

Aloe vera is a stemless plant that has fleshy leaves. The flesh of the leaves have a gel like consistency and is used to treat skin and hair problems, gut problems, and also aids weight loss.It has antioxidants that help detoxify and clean your body, boosts metabolism, and vitamins that help in proper functioning of the body.

Herbal (Ayurved) Technique Weight Loss

Where To Buy Aloe Vera?

You can buy aloe vera extract in pharmacy, ayurveda stores, supermarkets, or online. You can also grow an aloe vera plant (not wild) for topical applications.

How To Take Aloe Vera?

You can take 1-2 teaspoons of aloe vera extract every day. Or you can scoop out the aloe vera gel from the leaf and mix it with your morning juice or smoothie.

Aloe Vera Weight Loss Recipe

Ingredients

- 1 teaspoon aloe vera gel
- 1 cup water

How To Prepare

1. Mash the aloe vera gel using the back of a spoon.
2. Add water and stir well.

Benefits

Drinking this water every morning will keep your skin and hair healthy. It will also keep your digestive system healthy and promote quick weight loss.

Precautions

Do not use the gel of a wild aloe vera plant for consumption or topical application.

10. Cinnamon For Weight Loss

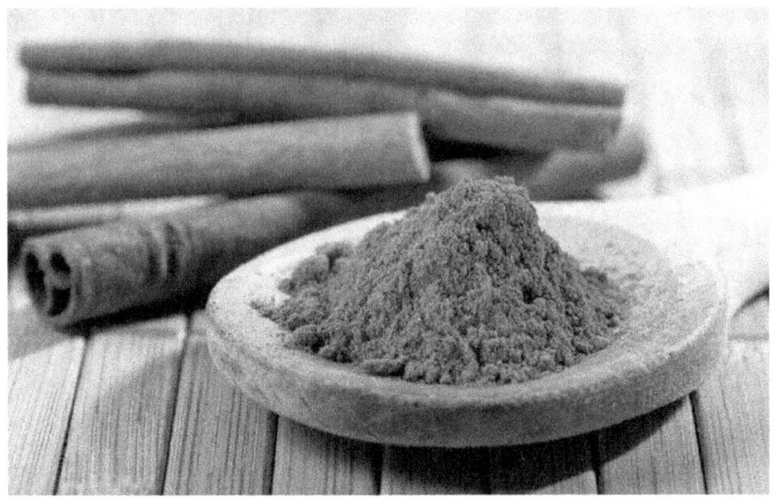

A popular Indian spice, it has both a sweet and strong flavor. Cinnamon helps quicken your metabolism. Cinnamon helps regulate blood sugar. It also plays a vital role in reducing blood sugar, LDL cholesterol, and triglycerides. With its benefits, it becomes an ideal condiment for those with diabetes. Cinnamon can also boost your glucose metabolism, which helps improve blood sugar regulation.

Where To Buy Cinnamon?

You can buy cinnamon at any Indian store, supermarket, or online.

How To Take Cinnamon?

You can take 1-2 teaspoons of cinnamon in powdered form or 1 cinnamon bark soaked in water overnight.

Drink cinnamon infused water first thing in the morning every day for four weeks to get desired results.

Cinnamon Tea Weight Loss Recipe

Ingredients

- 1 teaspoon cinnamon powder
- 1 cup water

How To Prepare

1. Bring a cup of water to a boil.
2. Add the cinnamon powder and let the water boil for 2-3 minutes more.
3. Strain the cinnamon tea before drinking.

Benefits

Cinnamon helps to suppress appetite, lower bad cholesterol and accelerates the metabolic rate. The warm water helps to flush out all the toxins and support better bowel movement, thereby preventing bloating.

Precautions

Do not consume Cassia cinnamon for weight loss. Always opt for Ceylon cinnamon.

11. Cardamom For Weight Loss

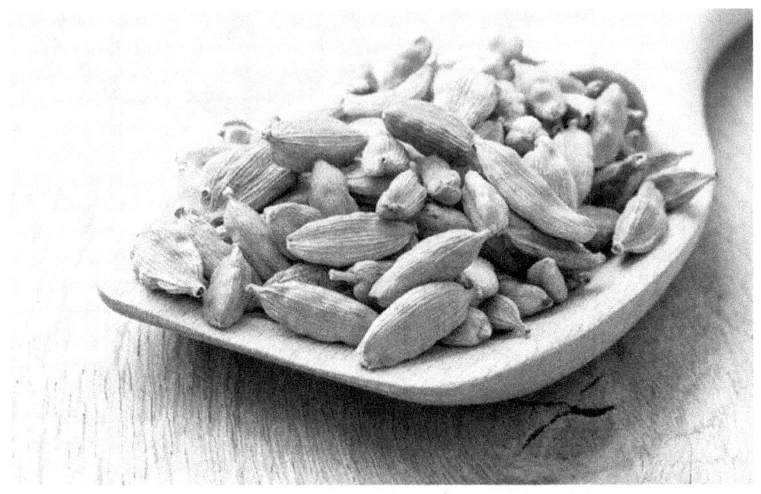

Another popular Indian spice with a unique flavor—cardamom or elaichi is a known thermogenic, which means that it burns fat for fuel to heat the body. Cardamom also boosts metabolism and in turn, helps the body burn more fat. It prevents the formation of gas that bloats up your stomach instantly. Cardamom has been widely used in the ancient Indian medical system—Ayurveda. Add a little elaichi or cardamom in your food to increase your body's metabolic rate.

Where To Buy Cardamom?

You can buy cardamom in any Indian store or supermarkets.

How To Take Cardamom?

You can take 1 teaspoon of cardamom powder once a day.

Herbal (Ayurved) Technique Weight Loss

Cardamom Weight Loss Recipe

Ingredients

- 1 teaspoon cardamom powder
- 1 cup water
- 1 tablespoon green tea leaves

How To Prepare

1. Bring a cup of water to a boil.
2. Add cardamom powder and let it boil for 2 minutes more.
3. Turn off the flame and add green tea leaves.
4. Let it steep for 5 minutes.
5. Strain the tea and stir well before drinking.

Benefits

Green tea is a metabolism booster and helps to flush out the toxins. Cardamom increases the internal body temperature, which helps to melt the extra body fat. This drink is a clear winner when it comes to losing weight.

Precautions

Do not use too much cardamom as it may lead to diarrhea and vomiting.

12. Garlic For Weight Loss

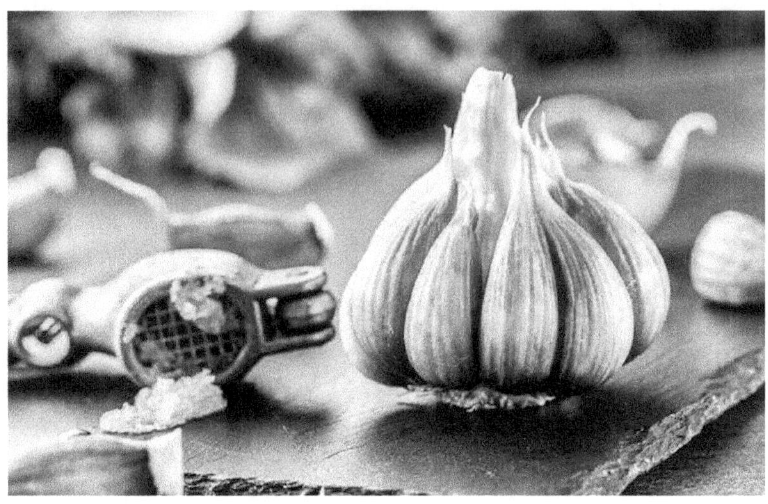

This herb comes with magical healing properties, which helps in treating cardiovascular conditions, improves your immune system and curing common cold to even fighting the fatal cancer! Recent research has shown that this magical herb can melt the fat in your waistline. Garlic contains a unique compound called allicin that suppresses hunger pangs and boosts metabolism.

Where To Buy Garlic?

You can buy garlic at the supermarket.

How To Take Garlic?

You can have one clove of garlic every day for best results. You can also include garlic in your daily recipes to add taste, flavor, and lose weight.

Herbal (Ayurved) Technique Weight Loss

Garlic Weight Loss Recipe

Ingredients

- 1 clove garlic
- 1 cup water
- Juice of ½ a lime

How To Prepare

1. Use a mortar and pestle to mash the garlic clove.
2. Add it to a cup of water.
3. Add lime juice, stir well, and drink at one go.

Benefits

The lime juice helps to cut the pungent smell and taste of the garlic. Limes are also rich in vitamin C that help boost the metabolism. Garlic helps to lower cholesterol, improves heart health, has anti-cancer properties, and aids weight loss by keeping your hunger pangs at bay.

Precautions

Do not consume too many garlic as the pungent smell is not easy to get rid of. It can also overheat your body and cause nausea and diarrhea.

13. Cayenne Pepper For Weight Loss

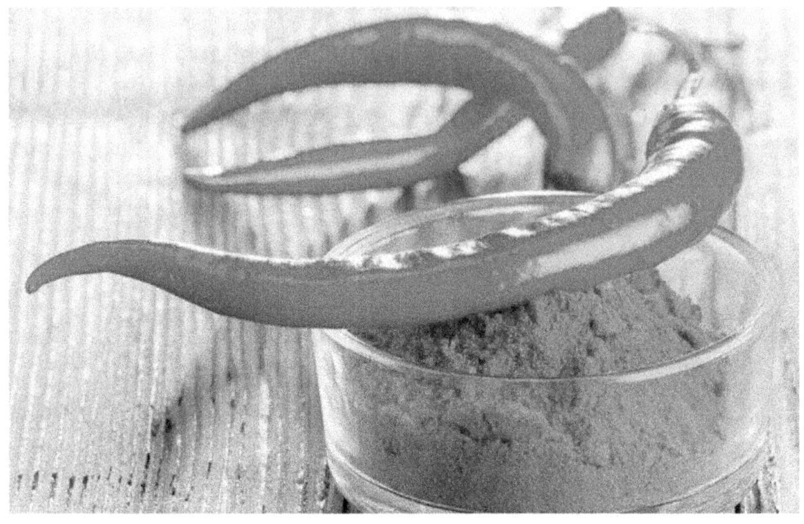

The main ingredient in Beyonce's famous **master cleanse diet**, Cayenne Pepper is rich in capsaicin, the compound that gives pepper its heat. As a known thermogenic, capsaicin stimulates the body to burn fat to create heat. It has been known to dissolve fat tissue and decrease the intake of calories. Cayenne Pepper also helps lower blood fat levels.

Where To Buy Cayenne Pepper?

You can buy cayenne pepper from any local supermarket.

How To Take Cayenne Pepper?

Take a ¼ teaspoon of cayenne pepper with your juice or smoothie twice a day.

Herbal (Ayurved) Technique Weight Loss

Cayenne Pepper Weight Loss Recipe

Ingredients

- ¼ teaspoon cayenne pepper
- 1 lime
- 1 cup water

How To Prepare

1. Squeeze out the juice of a lime into a glass.
2. Add a cup of water and ¼ teaspoon of cayenne pepper.
3. Stir well before drinking.

Benefits

The spiciness of cayenne pepper is perfectly balanced by the lime's acidic taste. Both the ingredients aid weight loss by boosting metabolism and burning body fat.

Precautions

Do not use too much of cayenne pepper to lose weight quickly. It will only lead to stomach upset, dizziness, and vomiting.

14. Black Pepper For Weight Loss

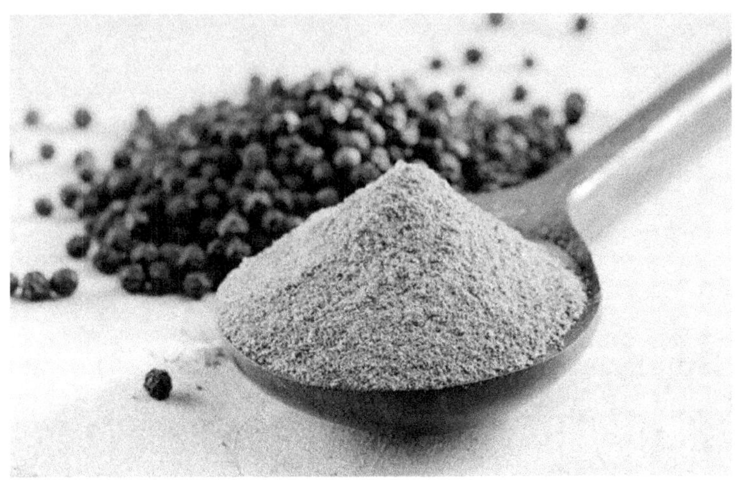

When we are speaking of pepper, let's not forget black pepper. A cousin of the Cayenne Pepper, the Black pepper is rich in piperine. Piperine is what gives black pepper its characteristic flavor. One of its characteristics is to inhibit the creation of fat cells, which help reduce weight. You can combine Black and Cayenne Pepper to speed up the fat burning process.

Where To Buy Black Pepper?

You can buy black pepper at any local supermarket.

How To Take Black Pepper?

You can either chew 5 black peppercorns per day or add it in your juice or food recipes.

Black Pepper Weight Loss Recipe

Ingredients

- ¼ teaspoon freshly ground black pepper
- ½ teaspoon honey
- 1 cup warm water

How To Prepare

1. Add 1 teaspoon honey and ¼ teaspoon black pepper to a cup of warm water.
2. Stir well before drinking.

Benefits

Black pepper aids weight loss by preventing fat cell proliferation and honey helps to boost the immunity and maintain a healthy gut. This drink helps to flush out the toxins from the body and gives you a clear skin and toned body when consumed regularly.

Precautions

Over consumption of black pepper may cause edema, stomach upset, and respiratory problems.

15. Ginger For Weight Loss

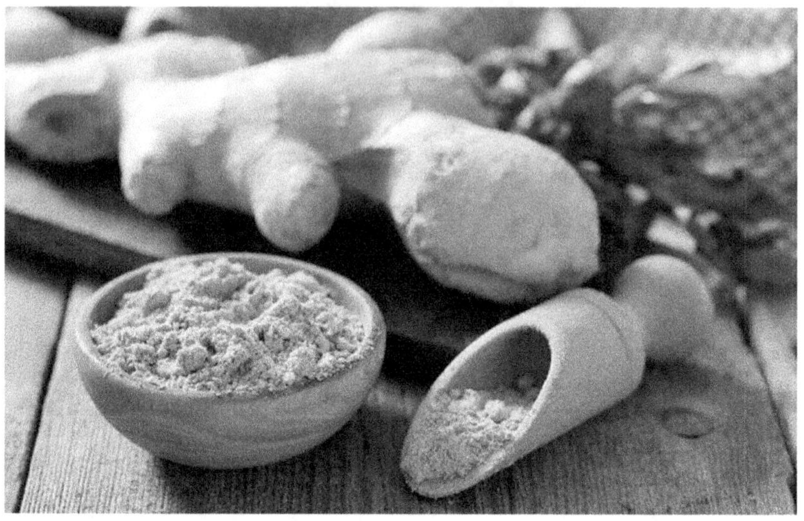

Ginger boosts metabolism by 20% that speeds up calorie burning process. Include little pieces of this herb in your dish and see how it fights obesity. It can also be used to treat a sore throat and a number of other conditions. It has antioxidant and anti-inflammatory properties that soothe the intestines. Ginger is also shown to have active appetite-suppressant characteristics, which ensure that you don't gorge on food.

Where To Buy Ginger?

You can buy ginger at any supermarket.

How To Take Ginger?

You can chew ½ inch ginger root or add it to your juice, smoothies or food recipes.

Herbal (Ayurved) Technique Weight Loss

Ginger Tea Weight Loss Recipe

Ingredients

- ½ inch ginger
- 1 teaspoon honey
- 1 cup water

How To Prepare

1. Bring a cup of water to a boil.
2. Use a mortar and pestle to crush the ginger root.
3. Add the crushed ginger root to the boiling water.
4. Let it boil for 2 minutes more.
5. Turn off the flame and add honey.
6. Strain and stir well before drinking.

Benefits

Ginger helps to improve gut health, flushes out toxins from the colon, prevents throat infections, and helps to melt fat. Honey balances the strong flavor of ginger, adds to the sweetness of the drink and boosts the immune system.

Precautions

Do not consume too much ginger as it may lead to nausea, gas, and stomach upset.

16. Cumin For Weight Loss

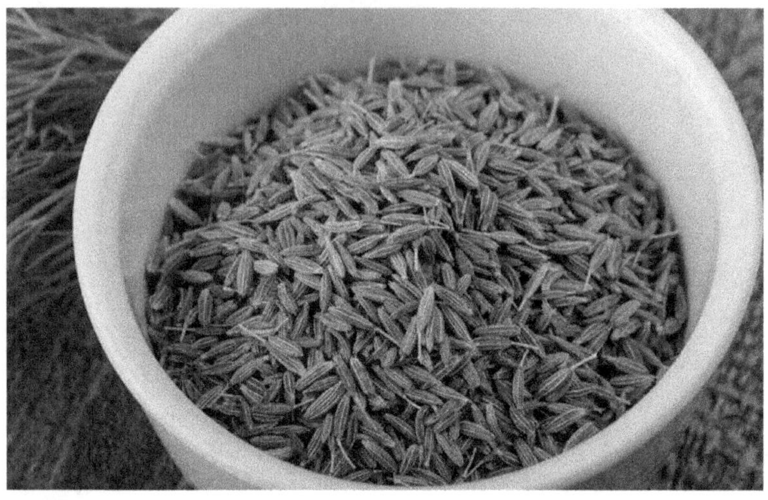

Cumin or Jeera is another popular spice that is used in almost every recipe in Indian cuisine. It helps the body get the required energy and is an excellent digestive. It is this digestive property that makes cumin an effective agent for weight loss.

Where To Buy?

You can buy cumin seeds at any Indian store or a local supermarket.

How To Take?

Take 2 teaspoons of cumin seeds soaked in water or 1 teaspoon cumin seed powder in juices or food recipes.

Cumin Weight Loss Recipe

Ingredients

- 2 teaspoons cumin seeds
- 1 cup water
- ½ teaspoon honey powder

How To Prepare

1. Soak the cumin seeds in water overnight.
2. Heat the water till it becomes warm.
3. Strain the water and add honey.
4. Stir well before drinking.

Benefits

Cumin seeds are extremely helpful in keeping good gut health. It also helps to sleep better, reduces the risk of respiratory disorders, common cold, anemia, and skin disorders. Honey is an antibacterial agent and helps to flush out the toxins. This drink can act as a magic potion if consumed regularly.

Precautions

Consuming cumin seeds in excess can cause bloating, diarrhea, and bowel spasms.

17. Dandelions For Weight Loss

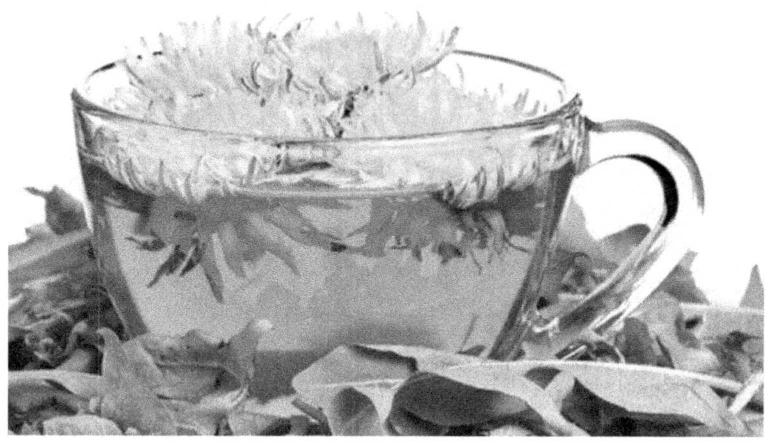

Dandelions aren't just beautiful; they are edible as well. In fact, they are loaded with nutrients. Dandelions have shown to slow down the digestive process. This ensures that you feel full for a longer time, which in turn ensures that you don't have too much to eat too often. Dandelions are rich in dietary fiber, antioxidants, minerals and Vitamin K1. They also contain beta-carotene, which attacks free radicals and helps protect your liver.

Where To Buy?

You can buy dandelion online or from Ayurveda stores.

How To Take?

You can take 1-2 teaspoons of dandelion or 1 dandelion pill with a full glass of water.

Dandelion Weight Loss Recipe

Ingredients

- 1 teaspoon dandelion
- 1 cup water

How To Prepare

1. Bring a cup of water to a boil.
2. Add the dandelion and let it boil for 2-3 minutes.
3. Strain and let it cool for few minutes before drinking.

Benefits

Dandelions are rich in fiber; it prevents absorption of fat molecules. The antioxidants help scavenge the harmful oxygen radicals and flush out the toxins.

Precautions

Do not use it until your doctor gives you a thumbs up. Avoid using during pregnancy.

18. Turmeric For Weight Loss

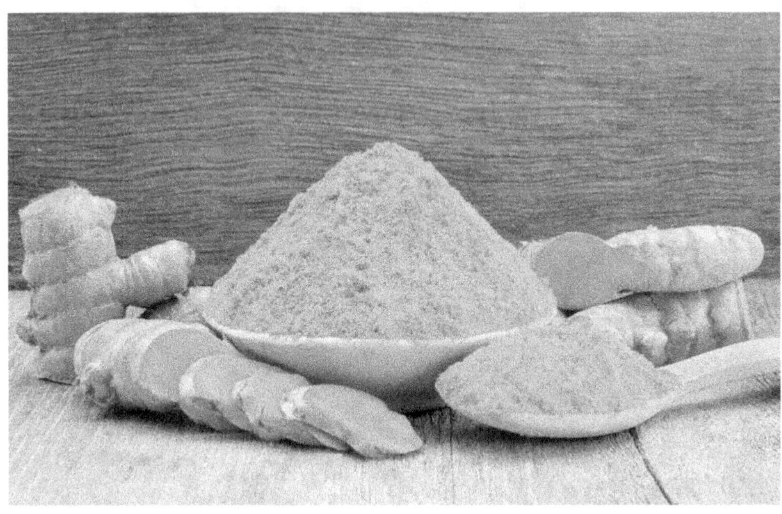

Turmeric, a bright yellow pigmented root is a native to Southern Asia. It has been used as a medicine in India for centuries. Curcumin, a compound responsible for turmeric's bright color, is also responsible for melting fat. Turmeric helps to lower bad cholesterol levels in the blood and helps to reduce inflammation.

Where To Buy?

You can buy turmeric in any Indian grocery store.

How To Take?

Chew ½ inch turmeric root or ½ – 2 teaspoons turmeric powder per day.

Turmeric Weight Loss Recipe

Ingredients

- ½ inch turmeric root
- 1 cup warm water
- ½ lime juice

How To Prepare

1. Use a mortar and pestle to crush the turmeric root.
2. Add it to a cup of warm water.
3. Add lime juice.
4. Stir well before drinking.

Benefits

It promotes rapid weight loss, improves gut and skin health. It prevents microbial infections, helps to heal wounds, and reduces pain.

Precautions

Consuming turmeric in excess can cause nausea, increased menstrual flow, and low blood pressure.

19. Rosemary For Weight Loss

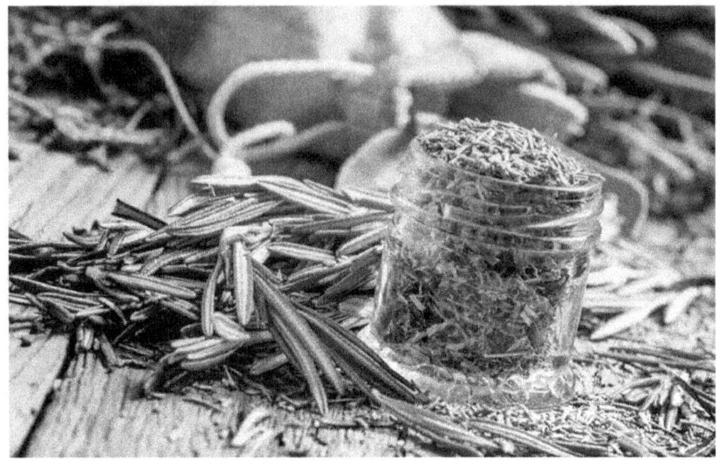

Rosemary is a perennial herb with green needle-like leaves. It is commonly used in food recipes, and its tea helps to reduce weight. Rosemary is a rich source of the enzyme lipase. Lipase is responsible for breaking down the fat molecules. Rosemary also contains fiber, which prevents fat absorption and keeps you full for longer hours.

Where To Buy?

You can buy rosemary from any local supermarket, pharmacy or online.

How To Take?

400 mg rosemary tablets thrice a day. You can also use fresh or dried rosemary in food.

Herbal (Ayurved) Technique Weight Loss

Rosemary Weight Loss Recipe

Ingredients

- 1 teaspoon fresh rosemary
- 1 cup water

How To Prepare

1. Bring a cup of water to a boil.
2. Turn the flame off and add rosemary.
3. Let it steep for 5-7 minutes.
4. Strain and drink.

Benefits

Rosemary improves digestion and boosts metabolism. It also helps to flush out the toxins from the colon and prevents bloating.

Precautions

Do not consume rosemary in excess as it may cause diarrhea and nausea. Avoid during pregnancy.

20. Gotu Kola For Weight Loss

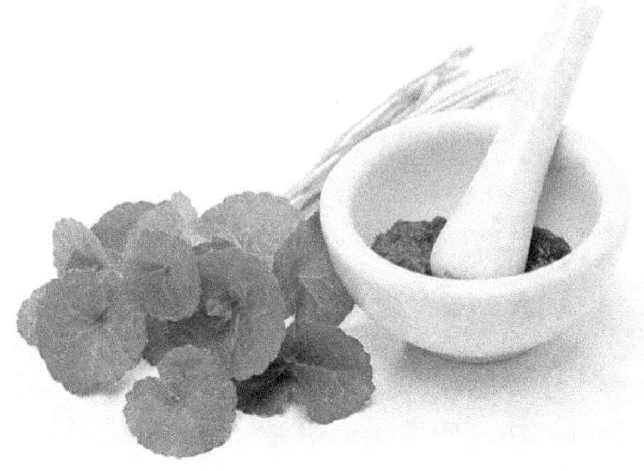

Gotu kola, also known as CENTELLA ASIATICA, has been used in Ayurveda and Chinese medicine since ages. It is extremely helpful in treating stress, depression, anxiety, Alzheimer's, improves memory and blood circulation. Gotu kola can also be consumed to prevent urinary tract infection, common cold, influenza, and tuberculosis.

Where To Buy?

You can buy Gotu kola in any Ayurveda store or online.

How To Take?

Take 1-2 teaspoons of Gotu kola per day.

Gotu Kola Weight Loss Recipe

Ingredients

- 1-2 teaspoons of Gotu kola

- 1 cup water

- 1 teaspoon honey

How To Prepare

1. Add Gotu kola to a cup of water and let it steep for 3 minutes.

2. Add honey and stir well before drinking.

Benefits

Stress is one of the factors that lead to weight gain. Gotu kola brings down stress, anxiety, and depression, which in turn stimulates the "feel-good" hormone. This indirectly leads to weight loss. You will feel more active and energetic. Honey is loaded with antioxidants and has antibacterial properties. It helps to flush out toxins and maintain a healthy gut.

Precautions

Consuming more than the recommended dose may cause drowsiness, stomach pain, and fever.

21. Neem For Weight Loss

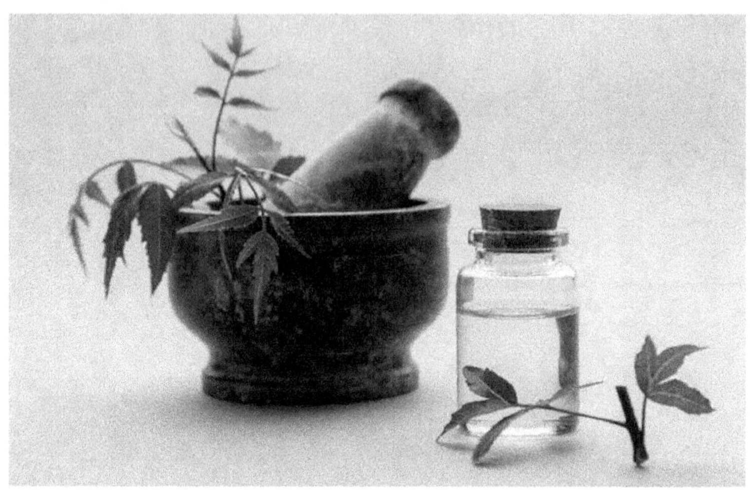

Neem, a medicinal tree, is native to India, Bangladesh, Pakistan, and Sri Lanka. It mainly grows in the tropical and subtropical regions. Its leaves, branches, and fruits contain medicinal properties and have been used since ages to treat many health conditions.

Where To Buy?

You can buy neem from any Ayurveda store, pharmacy or online. You could even pluck a few fresh leaves from the neem tree.

How To Take?

Chew 4-5 tender neem leaves per day or consume 1 teaspoon neem extract per day.

Herbal (Ayurved) Technique Weight Loss

Neem Weight Loss Recipe

Ingredients

- 4-5 neem leaves
- 1 cup water

How To Prepare

1. Use a mortar and pestle to crush the neem leaves.
2. Add it to a cup of water.
3. Stir well before drinking.

<u>Benefits</u>

Neem leaves have antimicrobial, anti-inflammatory, and antioxidant properties. It improves circulation and flushes out toxins from the body. It also helps to maintain good gut health. Neem leaves aid weight loss by reducing inflammation and boosting the metabolism.

<u>Precautions</u>

Over consumption of neem can cause stomach upset, heartburn, vomiting, and headache.

22. Fenugreek Seeds For Weight Loss

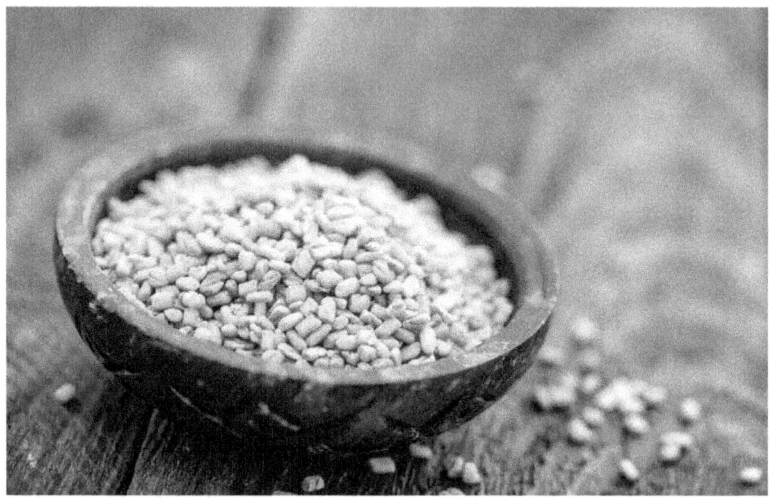

Fenugreek seeds, also known as Chandrika, Greek clover, and Methi, is native to western Asia, Mediterranean, and southern Europe. It is widely used to treat inflammation, constipation, obesity, polycystic ovarian disease, and helps to lower cholesterol.

Where To Buy?

You can buy fenugreek seeds from any Indian grocery store or online.

How To Take?

2 teaspoon fenugreek seeds per day with 1 cup water.

Weight Loss Recipe

Ingredients

- 2 teaspoons fenugreek seeds
- 1 cup water

How To Prepare

1. Soak 2 teaspoons of fenugreek seeds in a cup of water overnight.
2. Strain and drink the water first thing in the morning.

<u>Benefits</u>

It boosts metabolism, prevents obesity triggered by stress and inflammation, flushes out toxins from the colon, and reduces the risk of PCOD.

<u>Precautions</u>

Avoid using during pregnancy.

23. Mustard Seeds For Weight Loss

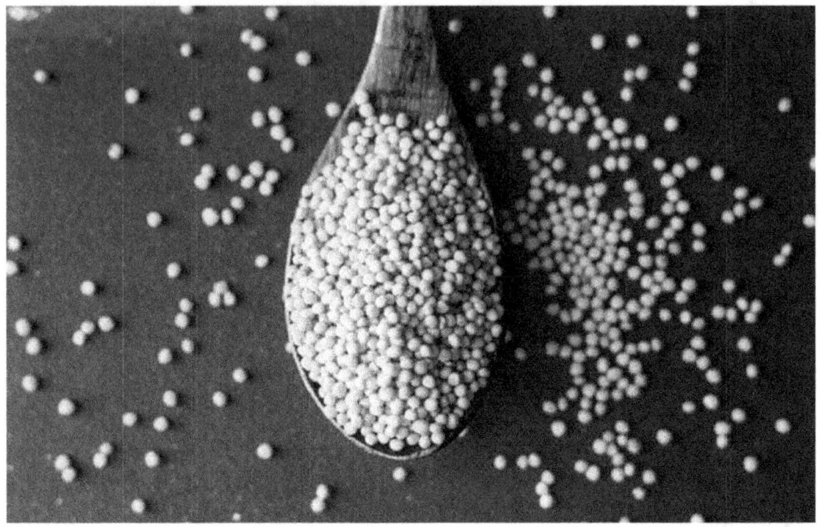

Mustard seeds are black or yellowish white seeds of the mustard plant. It mostly grows in India, Nepal, Hungary, Canada, and USA. It is mostly used in Indian curries, as a condiment, and salad dressing. These are low carbs and calories and are rich in vitamins such as vitamin B12, folate, thiamin, and niacin. It is also rich in omega-3-fatty acids and helps to lower the bad cholesterol levels.

Where To Buy?

You can buy mustard seeds in any local grocery store or supermarket.

How To Take?

You can consume mustard seeds in your food or as a low-calorie salad dressing.

Mustard Weight Loss Recipe

Ingredients

- 1 teaspoon mustard seed
- 1 teaspoon olive oil
- 1 teaspoon lime juice

How To Prepare

1. Soak the mustard seeds in water for 30 minutes.
2. Use a mortar and pestle to grind the seeds.
3. Add olive oil and lime juice to the ground mustard seeds.
4. Mix well and use it as a salad dressing.

Benefits

This low-calorie salad dressing is full of flavor and adds a zing to your salad. It is high in fiber and therefore will keep your hunger pangs at bay. The healthy fats in the seeds prevent inflammation. This, in turn, prevents inflammation-induced weight gain.

Precautions

Avoid consuming too much mustard seeds as it may cause heartburn and stomach upset.

24. Coriander Seeds For Weight Loss

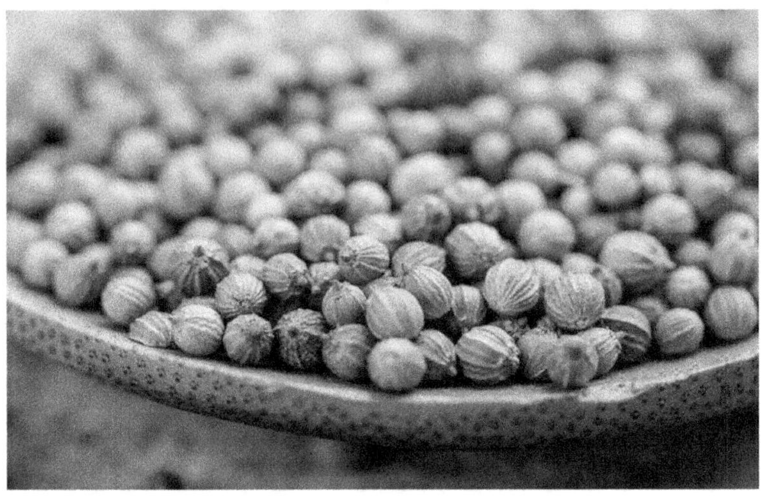

This aromatic spice is regularly used in Indian, Bangladeshi, and Pakistani cuisine. Coriander seeds are harvested from the plant when the seeds become brown. It is loaded with antioxidants, healthy fats, and minerals such as copper, potassium, zinc, calcium, and magnesium. It is also rich in vitamin C which boosts immunity.

Where To Buy?

You can buy coriander seeds or coriander powder in any Indian grocery store.

How To Take?

You can consume it as a spice in a curry or have 2 teaspoon coriander seeds soaked water in the morning.

Herbal (Ayurved) Technique Weight Loss

Coriander Weight Loss Recipe

Ingredients

- 2 teaspoon coriander seeds
- 1 cup water
- ½ teaspoon cinnamon powder

How To Prepare

1. Soak the coriander seeds in a cup of water overnight.
2. Strain the water in the morning.
3. Add cinnamon powder and let it steep for 10 minutes.
4. Strain before drinking.

Benefits

Coriander seeds are highly beneficial for proper digestion, absorption, and helps to maintain proper bowel movement. This, in turn, keeps the metabolism firing and burns the calories consumed. Cinnamon also aids weight loss by preventing fat cell proliferation.

Precautions

Avoid during pregnancy or before a surgery.

25. Fennel Seeds For Weight Loss

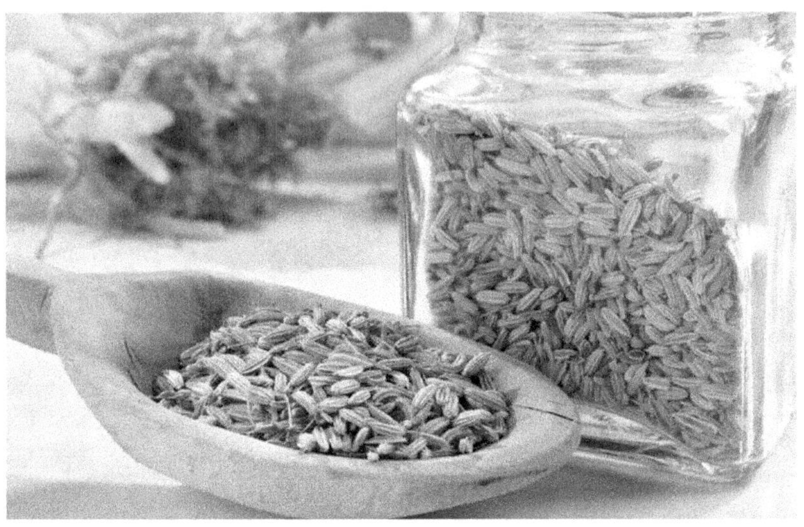

Fennel seeds are harvested from the fennel plant, which belongs to the carrot family. It is widely used as a culinary spice and also has medicinal uses. It has a sweet taste and helps in proper digestion. It is rich in antioxidants, dietary fiber, vitamins, and minerals.

Where To Buy?

You can buy fennel seeds at any Indian grocery store.

How To Take?

2 teaspoon fennel seeds or 1 teaspoon fennel seed powder per day.

Fennel Weight Loss Recipe

Ingredients

- 2 teaspoon fennel seeds
- 1 cup water

How To Prepare

1. Soak the fennel seeds in a cup of water overnight.
2. Strain the water before drinking in the morning.

Benefits

Fennel seeds are rich in dietary fiber and therefore prevents fat absorption by binding to the fat molecules. It is also rich in antioxidants that help to flush out the toxins and prevents bloating. It eases constipation problems by absorbing water throughout the digestive system.

Precautions

Consuming too much fennel seeds may cause diarrhea and nausea.

www.ingramcontent.com/pod-product-compliance
Lightning Source LLC
Chambersburg PA
CBHW060813260726
48660CB00002B/917